Prescription Drugs and Nutrition

D0645968

Prescription Drugs and Nutrition

Elizabeth Somer, MA, RD

Publisher: Robert H. Garrison, Jr., MA, RPh

Editor In Chief: Elizabeth Somer, MA, RD

Managing Editor: Lisa M. Moye

Editorial Director: Janet L. Haley

Art Director: Scott Mayeda

Production Directors: Jeff Elkind, Irene Villa

Copy Editors: Norma Trost Foor, Jean Forsythe, Mary Houser, Stephen C. Schneider, R. H. Garrison, Sr., RPh

Cover Design: Stefanko & Hetz, Jeff Elkind

Photography: Bob and Irene Nishihira, Carlsbad, CA

Illustration: Walter Stuart

Copyright © 1986 by Health Media of America, Inc.

For information regarding volume purchase discounts contact:
Health Media of America, Inc.
11300 Sorrento Valley Road, Suite 250
San Diego, CA 92121

Printed in the United States of America.

ISBN 0-937325-01-5

Contents

Introduction

Introduction

Prescription Drugs and Nutrition is a reference guide for individuals taking prescription medications or non-prescription medications, called Over-The-Counter (OTC) medications.

Section One provides information on how medications might affect nutritional status and health. Individuals who might have a greater risk for developing nutritional deficiencies and malnutrition are identified in Section Two.

The nutritional side effects of specific medications are discussed in Section Three. In this section, both OTC medications and prescription drugs are listed in alphabetical order. Tables and graphs provide additional information on the effect of medications on nutrition, as well as general dietary recommendations. In Section Four, the way that food affects the action and effectiveness of different medications is discussed.

Appendix A is a special section on the influence of vitamin B_6 on mood and temperament. Refer to Appendix B for common symptoms of nutritional deficiencies and refer to Appendix C for dietary sources of nutrients that might be deficient in the diet. In Appendix D, specific formulas are suggested for vitamin-mineral supplementation to meet the unique nutritional needs of people taking certain medications. The information in this book is provided as a guide to medication-induced nutrient deficiencies.

Vitamin-mineral supplementation to counteract medication-induced nutritional deficiencies should be done under the supervision of a physician.

1
Prescription Drug-Nutrient Interactions

The Changing Role Of Medications In The United States

Most people believe that certain medications have the power to cure, heal, and provide a sense of well-being. The medicine men of primitive cultures combined the powers of magic, drugs, and herbs to cure the emotional, physical, and mental ailments of their people. Industrialized countries invest billions of dollars in the advancement of medical technology. Whether a person's roots are in a primitive society or an advanced society, the belief in the power of certain medicines is a primary force in health care.

The types of medications available and their regulation have changed since 1900. Our parents or grandparents suffered and died from acute infectious diseases. Influenza, tuberculosis, and pneumonia were the plagues of that era. Lack of regulation and "patent medicines" in the late 1800s and early 1900s meant the consumer was not protected against fraud, misrepresentation, or dangerous or harmful products. If a patient "felt good" when taking a medication it probably contained cocaine, opium, morphine, heroin, or alcohol. Some medications had high alcohol contents and were sold in taverns.

1

Times have changed. People in the United States today do not die from influenza as they did in the early 1900s. Individuals also are protected by regulations governing the contents, purity, and effectiveness of medications. In contrast to the acute infectious diseases of our ancestors, the diseases that occur in modern society are the chronic, degenerative diseases: cardiovascular disease, cancer, diabetes, and hypertension. In addition, disorders that were unmanageable, such as epilepsy and certain behavioral disorders, can now be controlled with medications.

In an attempt to counteract the rising cost of health care in this country people are exploring self-help approaches to the prevention and treatment of disease. Sales of non-prescription medications and vitamin-mineral supplements reflect this trend. Every year, Americans spend over $650 million on more than 100,000 different non-prescription medications.[1]

The widespread use of prescription and non-prescription medications has contributed to interest in the interactions between individual medications and the interactions between diet and medications. It is now recognized that long-term use of certain medications might pose serious concerns about a person's nutritional status. In turn, the nutritional status of an individual can affect the desired outcome of the therapy.

How Medications Influence Nutritional Status

Prescription and non-prescription medications can affect a person's nutritional status in several ways. Medications can increase and decrease appetite, alter the absorption of nutrients in the intestine, affect how

Table 1	The Effects of Medications on Nutritional Status

Alteration of food intake.
    Changes in appetite.
    Changes in sense of taste and smell.
    Decrease in salivary secretion.
    Gastric irritation.
    Nausea and vomiting.
Alteration of nutrient absorption.
    Luminal Effects
        Changes in gastrointestinal pH.
        Changes in gastrointestinal motility.
        Changes in bile acid activity.
        Formation of drug-nutrient complexes.
    Mucosal Effects
        Inactivation of absorptive enzyme systems.
        Damage to gastrointestinal mucosal cells.
Alteration of nutrient metabolism and utilization.
Alteration of nutrient excretion.

nutrients are used within the body, and increase the excretion of nutrients. *(Table 1)*

Medications And Increased Appetite

Some medications cause an increase in appetite, food intake, and even cause cravings for specific foods, especially sweets. Medications that increase appetite cause concern because of the potential for obesity and its relation to the degenerative diseases: cardiovascular disease, cancer, diabetes, and hypertension. Certain tricyclic antidepressants, such as amitriptyline (Elavil), are known to have such an effect.[2]

Other medications that might increase appetite are chlordiazepoxide (Librium), benzodiazepines, phenothiazines, lithium carbonate, diazepam (Valium), and the antihistamine cyproheptadine (Periactin).[2,3] This stimulation of appetite occurs even at low doses. At high doses, these medications can cause lethargy and a general disinterest in food and eating. Malnutrition and weight loss can result.

Medications And Reduced Appetite

Medications that diminish appetite also cause special concerns. Loss of appetite (anorexia) means a reduced food and nutrient intake and the potential for nutrient deficiencies, malnutrition, and loss of lean body mass. This increases the risk for people who are already borderline for nutritional deficiencies. The chemotherapeutic medications used in the treatment of cancer can cause a reduction in appetite (anorexia) and weight loss by their side effects of nausea, vomiting, diarrhea, and dry or sore mouth and throat. Taste alterations that result from some medications such as clofibrate, lincomycin, griseofulvin, and some tranquilizers can reduce a person's interest in eating. *(Table 2)* A second adverse effect of this medication-induced anorexia is that the resultant malnutrition reduces the efficiency of the immune system and interferes with the body's ability to defend itself against disease. *(Table 4 and 5, page 8, 9)*

Medications can affect food intake by altering a person's mood. Eating behaviors are strongly influenced by a delicate balance of psychological and physiological factors. The behavioral side effects of certain medications can affect this balance and reduce a person's desire to eat. *(Table 3, page 7)*

Table 2   Drugs & Taste Abnormalities

Medication	Effect on Taste
Amphetamines	Decreased sweet sensitivity or Increased bitter sensitivity.
Anesthetics	
Eucaine	Decreased bitter and sweet sensitivity.
Amydrieaine	Decreased bitter and sweet sensitivity.
Amylocaine	With high intake, loss of salt detection, decreased bitter sensitivity.
Isococaine and tropacocaine	Decreased sweet sensitivity.
Benzocaine	Increased sour sensitivity.
Amethocaine	Increased bitter sensitivity. Decreased sweet sensitivity.
Lidocaine	Decreased salt and sweet sensitivity.
Anti-thyroid agents	
Methimazole	Decreased sensitivity
Methylthiouracil	Decreased sensitivity.
Bentyl	Decreased sensitivity.
Choloxin	Changes in taste perception.
Clindamycin HCl hydrate	Bitter aftertaste
Clofibrate	Decreased sensitivity; unpleasant aftertaste.
Dinitrophenol	Loss of salt taste; general hypogeusia.
5-Fluorouracil	Some alterations in bitter and sour sensitivity. Increased sweet sensitivity.
Griseofulvin	Decreased sensitivity.
Insulin	Decreased sweet and salt sensitivity, with prolonged use.

(Continued on next page)

Table 2	Drugs & Taste Abnormalities *(Cont.)*
Medication	**Effect on Taste**
Lithium carbonate	Unpleasant taste.
Meprobamate	Decreased sensitivity.
Methicillin sodium	Aftertaste.
Oxyfedrine	Decreased sensitivity.
D-Penicillamine	General decrease in sensitivity.
Phenindione	Decreased sensitivity.
Phenytoin	Decreased sensitivity.
Probucol	Decreased sensitivity.
Propantheline bromide	Decreased sensitivity.

Medications are not the only way appetite is depressed in people who are ill. In many cases, it is not the medication but the illness that causes the anorexia. A loss of appetite is associated with the following illnesses:

- Acute bronchitis (inflammation of the bronchial tubes in the lungs)
- Acute cholecystitis (inflammation of the bile duct)
- Acute confusional psychosis
- Burns
- Fractures
- Generalized dermatitis or other dermatoses with severe itching
- Intestinal obstruction
- Oral candidiasis (a yeast infection of the mouth)
- Pneumonia (viral or bacterial)
- Other viral and bacterial infections *(Table 6 and 7, page 10)*

Table 3	Loss of Appetite: What to Do

If a medication causes a temporary loss of appetite, the following suggestions might improve food intake:

- Eat with friends or family whenever possible.
- Make food appetizing. Choose a variety of colors, textures, and aromas and serve food attractively.
- Create a pleasant atmosphere at the dining table. Use soft lights, quiet music, and brightly colored table accessories.
- Sip on fluids that provide calories (juices, milk-shakes, milk, or nectars).
- Have snacks by the bed at night (nuts, dried fruits, or candy).
- Place snacks throughout the house or keep non-sugary foods readily available, such as fresh or dried fruits, vegetables, or cottage cheese.
- Schedule small quantities of food to eat, i.e., two bites every hour or eat small meals frequently throughout the day.
- Eat when hungry, regardless of time.
- Exercise about one-half hour prior to a meal.
- Vary the diet and try new recipes.
- Use days when eating is enjoyable to catch up on nutrition.
- Take a multiple vitamin-mineral supplement with consent of your physician.
- If poor appetite persists, consult a physician.

Table 4	Taste Changes: What to Do
	If medications alter the taste of food or cause it to be bitter or tasteless try the following:

- Try highly seasoned and flavored foods.
- Avoid beef or pork, since these meats are the most likely to cause taste aversions.
- Prepare foods that look and smell appetizing.
- Try chicken, turkey, fish, eggs, and dairy products if red meat is not appealing. Avoid strong smelling fish.
- Acceptable foods might include: bland cheeses, cottage cheese, fresh fruits, gelatins, salads, ice cream, lettuce, or peanut butter.
- Pleasant smells might help, i.e., freshly baked bread or simmering soup.
- Brush the teeth before eating.
- Rely on other senses to provide a pleasurable atmosphere. Decorate the room and table, eat foods that provide a variety of colors and textures, include flowers on the table.
- If taste alterations persist, consult a physician.

Medications Might Affect Nutrient Absorption

Most medications and nutrients are absorbed in the small intestine and can interact with each other to impair the absorption of one or both.

Medications can interfere with nutrient absorption in numerous ways. Medications can bind to a nutrient in the intestinal tract and hinder its absorption; this occurs with mineral oil and the fat-soluble vitamins.[4-6] Medications can speed transit time of food and nutri-

Table 5	Nausea: What to Do

If a medications produces temporary nausea, try the following:

- Eat small meals frequently throughout the day.
- Avoid liquids at mealtimes. Drink fluids one hour before or after meals.
- Avoid sweets and fried or fatty foods.
- Eat slowly.
- Recruit family members, neighbors, and friends to help with shopping, preparation, and clean-up of meals.
- Chew food well.
- Eat dry foods, such as toast and crackers. These foods ease upset stomach, especially in the morning.
- Drink cold, clear liquids, such as apple juice, cranberry juice, or broth.
- Eat light meals, such as soup and crackers, before treatment, unless nausea results from radiation. In this case, refrain from eating for several hours prior to treatment.
- Avoid the kitchen if the smell of food produces nausea or vomiting.
- Do not lie down for at least two hours following a meal. Resting in a comfortable chair, however, is helpful for digestion.
- Take deep breaths or find other distractions to relieve nausea.
- If nausea is severe or persists, consult a physician.

ents and reduce the contact time between the absorptive intestinal wall and the essential vitamin or mineral.[6]

Table 6	Fullness and Bloating: What to Do
	If a medication causes a feeling of fullness or bloating try the following:

- Take meals without fluids. Drink fluids between meals.
- Avoid gas-forming foods, such as cabbage, dried beans and peas, or raisins.
- Eat and drink slowly.
- Choose foods that leave the stomach quickly, i.e., breads, cereals, fruits, juices, and vegetables.
- Avoid fatty foods.
- Eat small amounts of food at frequent intervals.
- When feeling full, stop eating for a short time.
- If fullness or bloating persists, consult a physician.

Medications can change the structure or function of a nutrient so that it becomes insoluble in the watery medium of the intestines and cannot be absorbed.

Table 7	Heartburn: What to Do
	If a medication causes temporary heartburn, try the following:

- Eat small quantities of food at frequent intervals.
- Do not homogenize, mince, or puree foods.
- Limit the use of alcohol, coffee, tea, and other caffeine-containing beverages.
- Avoid spicy, greasy, fried, or fatty foods.
- Avoid eating before bedtime.

Table 8	Classes of Medications that Cause Nutrient Malabsorption
	• Medications that affect intestinal motility, such as laxatives and cathartics.
	• Hypocholesterolemic medications, such as cholestyramine, clofibrate, and colestipol.
	• Some oral medications for diabetes.
	• Antibiotic medications, such as neomycin and tetracycline.
	• Anti-gout medications, such as colchicine.

Medications also can change the acidity of the intestinal tract and impair the absorption of nutrients.

Medications can physically or chemically block absorption sites on the intestinal wall or reduce the absorption capabilities of the intestinal lining.[6]

Medications can absorb or interfere with the bile salts so that dietary fat and the fat-soluble vitamins are poorly absorbed through the intestinal lining. Finally, medications can interfere with the functioning of the pancreas and its digestive enzymes that are required for the absorption of fat, protein, and carbohydrate. Neomycin reduces the absorption of dietary fat because it inhibits normal fat digestion.[4,7] *(Table 8)*

Medications That Might Affect How Nutrients Are Used In The Body

The effect of medications on how the body uses a nutrient is complicated. Some medications mimic the

11

shape of a vitamin, but do not have the same activity. In the body, these medications can be mistaken for the vitamin and can block the real vitamin from entering into metabolic reactions.

Other medications can bind to the active site on an enzyme where normally a vitamin or mineral would bind. The vitamin or mineral is excreted, the enzyme cannot function, and all body processes that depend on the enzyme are halted.

Vitamin B_6 is an example. This vitamin acts as an enzyme in several metabolic reactions that involve the breakdown, building, and alteration of proteins and their components. Certain medications might potentially bind to vitamin B_6 and keep it from its normal duties. Five categories of medications interfere with vitamin B_6: alcohol; hydrazine medications, such as hydralazine; medications for Parkinson's Disease, such as L-DOPA; medications for Wilson's Disease, such as D-Penicillamine; and oral contraceptives.[8]

A medication-induced vitamin B_6 deficiency does not produce obvious symptoms. However, physiological and psychological changes can develop when nutrients are at marginal levels.[8] Poor vitamin B_6 status is associated with an increased risk for cardiovascular disease, irregular sleep habits, irritability, lethargy, and a reduced ability to handle stress.[9]

Finally, medications can alter the amount and site of nutrient storage within the body. For example, oral contraceptives affect the distribution of vitamin B_{12} in the tissues.[4] *(Table 9)*

Table 9	Medications that Affect Vitamin B_{12} and Folic Acid Status		
	Achromycin	Klotrix	Percodan
	Aldoril	K-lyte	Septra
	Aldomet	K-tab	Slow K
	Bactrim	Micro-K	Sumycin
	Butazolidin	Macrodantin	Stelazine
	Dyazide	Medrol	Tagamet
	Donnatal	Oral Contraceptives	
	Deltasone	Premarin	

Medications Might Increase Excretion of Nutrients

Medications such as diuretics, laxatives, and cathartics can increase the excretion of nutrients. Medicine-induced mineral imbalances are the most common result of this loss. Minerals coexist in a delicate balance with each other. When a medication interferes with one mineral, it can upset the balance of other minerals as well. Since it is common for people to take more than one medication at a time, the combined effect can result in numerous changes in mineral status. *(Table 10, page 14)*

Summary

Prescription and non-prescription medications often aggravate a pre-existing nutrient deficiency. Poor dietary intake or malabsorption of dietary nutrients can

Table 10	Diarrhea: What to Do
	If a medication causes temporary diarrhea, try the following:

- Eat foods warm rather than hot. Higher temperatures increase transit time of foods in the intestines, making bowels looser.

- Avoid gas-producing foods, such as beans, cabbage, broccoli, cauliflower, chewing gum, soda, highly spiced foods, and too many sweets. Let carbonated drinks lose their fizzle before drinking. Avoid caffeine-containing foods such as coffee, tea, cola, and chocolate.

- Include potassium rich-foods, such as bananas, potatoes, or apricot or peach nectar in the diet.

- Dairy products aggravate diarrhea and might need to be avoided temporarily.

- Do not skip meals if possible.

- Eat low fiber foods, such as bananas, macaroni, and cheese.

- Avoid high fiber foods, such as whole grain breads and cereals, raw fruits and vegetables, popcorn, and nuts.

- Eat foods that contain pectin, such as applesauce, or grated apples.

- If diarrhea is severe or persists, consult a physician.

produce deficiencies that often go unnoticed. When a medication that interferes with nutrients is added to the person's daily intake these subtle deficiencies might be increased.

The extent that a medication influences a person's nutritional state depends on the following:

- the body's nutrient reserves
- age, size, and medical condition
- individual variations in absorption and excretion of nutrients
- the adequacy of dietary intake
- the amount and duration of medication therapy

When the body does not adapt or the diet is not sufficient to overcome the imbalances caused by medication therapy, progressive nutrient depletion might result.

2
Nutritional Deficiencies: Who is at Risk?

Marginal Deficiencies

Nutritional deficiency symptoms were traditionally associated with the classic diseases such as beri beri, scurvy, pellagra, and rickets. These diseases are caused by severe nutrient deficiencies. As diagnostic and research techniques advance, the effect on health of less severe marginal nutrient deficiencies is better understood. The interaction between medications and nutrition is now a concern because of the possibility of marginal deficiencies.

Some deficiency symptoms are not apparent and it is easy for a marginal state to go unnoticed. The obvious symptoms of a deficiency might be lethargy, irritability, poor concentration, or insomnia. These symptoms are blamed on age or the weather, when the cause might be poor nutritional status. Deficiencies could affect the immune system. These deficiencies also might affect the brain and central nervous system, which in turn affects mood, mental capacity, and other biological and psychological conditions.

Marginal nutrient deficiencies can alter the effectiveness of a medication. Most medications must be structurally changed before they can be excreted. This process requires enzymes and their associated vitamins

17

or minerals. Individuals with marginal deficiencies of one or more vitamins or minerals have an altered or diminished ability to metabolize certain medications.

A medication proceeds through two phases before it is excreted. Once absorbed into the body from the intestines, the major route of excretion for most medications is through the urine. The first phase of transformation requires any medication that is not water-soluble be converted to a water-soluble form in order to be transported to the kidneys for excretion. Several nutrients participate in the first phase of medication transformation. These include the following:

1. Vitamins: C, Riboflavin (B_2), Niacin, Pantothenic Acid
2. Minerals: Calcium, Copper, Iron, Magnesium, Zinc
3. Protein
4. Glycine

If one or more of these nutrients is in short supply, metabolism of a medication might be incomplete.[10] This might cause prolonged activity of the circulating medication or a variety of adverse side effects.

During the second phase of transformation the water-soluble medication is either altered in shape or combined with another substance. This transformation requires the following nutrients:

1. Vitamins: Niacin, B_{12}, Folic Acid, Pantothenic Acid
2. Amino Acids
3. Carbohydrates
4. Fatty Acids
5. Lipoic Acid

Again, if the body storage level of one or more of these nutrients is low, metabolism and excretion of a medication might be hindered.[10]

Although marginal nutritional deficiencies might not be life threatening, they do reduce the quality of life. Deficiencies interfere with the diet and exercise patterns that would improve the quality of life and reduce the likelihood of developing cardiovascular disease, diabetes, cancer, and hypertension. For these reasons, marginal deficiencies should not be ignored.

Who is at Risk?

Malnutrition is most likely to develop in people on long-term medication therapy. The elderly, children, alcoholics, and the chronically ill are the most vulnerable. However, nutritional deficiencies are a result of many factors, including the nutritional state of the individual prior to medication therapy. If nutritional status and dietary intake are good, medication-induced nutritional deficiencies are less likely. If the person, however, has a disease such as cancer; has lost more than 10% of ideal body weight; has a poor dietary intake, such as alcoholics and patients on chemotherapy for cancer; has a chronic disease of the gastrointestinal tract; or has increased nutritional requirements as a result of injury, major surgery, or infection the additional effects of medication on nutritional status might result in nutrient deficiencies.[11,12]

People in high risk groups should begin preventive or rehabilitation measures, such as the addition of nutritional supplements or changes in dietary pat-

Table 11	Medications Associated With Nutrient Deficiencies in the Elderly
Medical Condition	**Medication**
Cardiovascular Disease	Digitalis
Hypertension	Thiazides (i.e., hydrochlorothiazide) — Furosemide — Ethacrynic acid — Mercurial diuretics — Triamterene
Arthritis	Aspirin
Gout	Indomethacin Colchicine
Indigestion (Antacids)	Magnesium and aluminum hydroxide
Constipation (Laxatives)	Mineral oil, phenolphthalein
Insomnia/Anxiety (Sedatives)	Barbiturates

terns, and should monitor nutritional status while taking medications.

The Elderly

People in the United States over 65 years old account for 11% of the population or 25 million people.[13] The elderly are the primary users of prescription and non-prescription medications. Over 80% of this population consumes more than two medications daily[14] and 61% take non-prescription medications.[15] The elderly account for 25% of total medication expenditures.[16] *(Table 11)*

Even when they are not using medications, the elderly are at high risk for nutrient deficiencies. A combination of poor diet, disease, and reduced ability to absorb and use nutrients can result in malnutrition. Illness, a limited income, and reduced mobility can restrict access to food and its preparation. Special diets, reduced appetite, disinterest in food, oral and dental problems, and social isolation are all factors that interfere with adequate food and nutrient intake in the elderly. As a result, many people in this age group have serious nutrient deficiencies. The use of long-term or multiple medication therapies and the increased likelihood of errors during self-medication further jeopardize nutritional status.[17,18]

The most common cause of medication-induced malnutrition in the elderly is the misuse of non-prescription medications. Analgesics, laxatives, and antacids are the major classes of non-prescription medications used by this population. These medications can interfere with mineral absorption and excretion, which might cause deficiencies. *(Table 12, page 22)* These adverse side effects are of special concern in individuals who are marginally nourished or who are suffering from malnutrition prior to self-medication.

People Who Drink Alcohol in Excess

Alcohol is the number one cause of malnutrition in otherwise healthy people. The abuse of alcohol can cause loss of appetite and this reduced interest in food is partially attributed to nutritional deficiencies of the B vitamin thiamin, the trace mineral zinc, and

Table 12   Medications and Their Effect on Nutritional Status in the Elderly

Medication	Effect on Nutritional Status
1. Cardiac glycosides Digitalis	Anorexia, protein malnutrition, zinc and magnesium deficiency

Lipid-lowering agents
   Cholestyramine
   Colestipol
   Clofibrate
   Neomycin
	Deficiencies of the fat-soluble vitamins A, D, E, K; deficiencies of vitamin B_{12}, folic acid, iron, and calcium

2. Diuretics:
   Thiazides
   Furosemide
   Ethacrynic acid
	Potassium, zinc, and magnesium depletion

Trimaterene Mercurial diuretics	Folic acid and protein deficiency

3. Anti-inflammatory medications
   Aspirin
   Indomethacin
	Gastrointestinal blood loss and iron deficiency anemia

Colchicine	Poor absorption of vitamins
4. Antacids	Phosphate deficiency and osteomalacia

5. Laxatives:
   Mineral Oil
   Phenolphthalein
	Deficiencies of vitamins A, D, K;
	Potassium deficiency; multiple nutrient deficiencies, especially folic acid and vitamin D.

Table 13	Nutrients at Risk in Alcoholics	
Vitamins:		Thiamin (B_1)
		Riboflavin (B_2)
		Niacin
		Pyridoxine (B_6)
		Cobalamine (B_{12})
		Folic Acid
		Ascorbic Acid (C)
Minerals:		Magnesium
		Zinc
Electrolytes:		Sodium
		Potassium
		Chloride
Amino acids		
Fatty acids		

protein.[2] Nutritional deficiencies are also a secondary effect of alcohol-induced disorders such as inflammation of the stomach, intestines, or liver; lactose intolerance; and cirrhosis of the liver.[19]

Alcohol can damage the intestinal lining and reduce the absorption of nutrients that are consumed. Deficiencies of vitamin B_1 and folic acid are common in people who abuse alcohol.[20,22] However, deficiencies of almost any nutrient can result from alcohol abuse. *(Table 13)*

People With Chronic Diseases

Medication-induced nutritional deficiencies are more likely to develop in people with chronic diseases, such as cardiovascular disease, diabetes, cancer, hyperten-

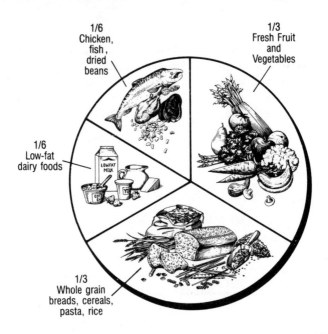

1/6
Chicken,
fish,
dried
beans

1/3
Fresh Fruit
and
Vegetables

1/6
Low-fat
dairy foods

1/3
Whole grain
breads, cereals,
pasta, rice

Graph 1. The Nutrient-Dense Diet
Limit the intake of butter, margarine, shortening, vegetable oils, fatty meats, and fatty dairy foods. Prepare foods by steaming, baking, poaching, or broiling.

sion, or epilepsy; disorders of the gastrointestinal tract; or behavioral disorders. This occurs because of the individual's long-term exposure to medications and the likelihood of multiple medication therapy.

Nutrient depletion, as a result of a disease or the medication therapy, is gradual and often does not become apparent until nutrient stores are exhausted. Since long-term treatment is likely to threaten a person's nutritional health, preventive measures, which include consumption of a nutritious diet *(Graph 1)* and supplementation, are essential.

Dosage also contributes to medication-induced malnutrition. A high dose of a medication taken for a long period of time is more likely to cause nutritional side effects than a low dose over a short period of time. This is also true of non-prescription medications such as laxatives and aspirin.

People With Increased Nutrient Needs Or Decreased Nutrient Intakes

People on weight control diets or restrictive diets; adolescents; women on oral contraceptives; and pregnant or lactating women are at risk for medication-induced nutritional deficiencies. These groups are likely to be marginally nourished because of restricted food intake, reliance on high calorie-low nutrient foods, or increased nutrient requirements. The effects of these diets, combined with the adverse nutritional effects of some medications, increases the potential for malnutrition.

3
Specific Medications and the Effect on Nutrition

Antacids

Antacids can cause nutritional deficiencies because people misuse these non-prescription medications. Antacids are frequently taken in excess to curb problems produced by the misuse of other dietary substances, such as alcohol or coffee, or by excessive eating.

Antacids that contain magnesium or aluminum hydroxide might interfere with the absorption of several nutrients. These antacids bind to dietary phosphates in the intestines and increase their excretion.[23] This upsets the delicate ratio of calcium to phosphorus that is necessary for normal calcium absorption and deposition into bone. Bone disorders might result.[24-26] This risk for bone disorders is further increased in the elderly who cannot absorb calcium well and who often consume inadequate amounts of calcium-rich foods in the diet.

Because antacids neutralize excess acid in the gastrointestinal tract they might interfere with the absorption of iron[27] and the B vitamins folic acid and B_{12}. The functions of folic acid and vitamin B_{12} are related. A deficiency of either vitamin results in anemia, which is a reduction in red blood cells, and a reduced ability to build and repair tissues.[28]

Table 14	The Nutritional Effects of Antacids	
	Nutritional Consequences	Type of Antacid
	Aluminum toxicity	Aluminum Hydroxide
	Folic acid malabsorption	Sodium Bicarbonate
	Magnesium overload	Magnesium Hydroxide
	Milk-alkali syndrome	Sodium Bicarbonate
	Phosphate depletion	Aluminum or Magnesium Hydroxide
	Sodium overload	Sodium Bicarbonate

Cimetidine (Tagamet), a medication that inhibits the secretion of stomach acid and is used in the treatment of ulcers, also reduces vitamin B_{12} absorption.[29]

The therapeutic effects of antacids depend on when they are taken. If aluminum hydroxide is taken to reduce gastric acidity, it should be taken two hours before or after a meal. Since there is no food in the stomach at this time, the antacid does not affect nutrient absorption and is less likely to cause nutrient deficiencies. When the same medication is used to rid the body of excess phosphates, it is taken with a meal. In this case, the antacid binds to dietary phosphorus and does not allow it to be absorbed. *(Table 14)*

Antibiotics

Antibiotics are important in the treatment of infections such as pneumonia, tuberculosis, and influenza, but these prescription medications have nutritional side effects. Some essential nutrients are produced by bacteria in the small and large intestines and are absorbed through the intestinal wall. Antibiotics disturb this normal bacterial growth and destroy the nutrient-producing bacteria. A deficiency of vitamin K can result.[30]

Tetracycline is an antibiotic that can inactivate the intestinal bacteria that manufacture vitamin K. This antibiotic also reduces vitamin C stores in the body.[31] Some minerals such as calcium and iron can reduce the effectiveness of tetracycline. (See page 51) Absorption of these minerals also is reduced and might result in a deficiency.[32,33]

Neomycin reduces the absorption of nutrients in several ways. This antibiotic changes the lining of the gastrointestinal tract so that it is less efficient at absorbing nutrients and binds bile and fat-soluble vitamins and inhibits their absorption. It also increases the excretion of nitrogen, sodium, potassium, and calcium; reduces the absorption of folic acid, iron, vitamin B_{12}, and vitamin K; and reduces the absorption of the sugars, sucrose and lactose.[34,37]

Other antibiotics are associated with reduced protein use, reduced utilization of folic acid and vitamin B_6, impaired use of amino acids, and malabsorption of vitamin B_{12}, calcium, and magnesium.[30]

Anticonvulsants

Anticonvulsant medications are used to control epileptic seizures and to prevent or treat seizures that result from neurosurgical procedures or head injures. Long-term anticonvulsant therapy with phenytoin (Dilantin), phenobarbital, primidone, or carbamazepine might cause rickets and osteomalacia.[38,53]

These medications inhibit the biological manufacture of vitamin D. This vitamin acts like a hormone to regulate calcium absorption from the intestines and deposition and removal from the bones. A vitamin D deficiency, even with adequate calcium intake, will cause bone degeneration. It is recommended that individuals who take anticonvulsant medications also take a vitamin D supplement that contains 400 to 800 IU of the fat-soluble vitamin.[10,39]

The anticonvulsant medications also are associated with anemia. This anemia is caused by a deficiency of folic acid and vitamin K and is characterized by frequent hemorrhage. However, if large doses of folic acid are given to counteract low blood levels, a possible underlying deficiency of vitamin B_{12} might go unnoticed.[40,41] To avoid these deficiencies, a daily supplement of vitamin K, folic acid, and vitamin B_{12} might be necessary.[42] Since folic acid in high doses can interfere with the action of some anticonvulsants, such as phenytoin, supplements should not be taken without prior approval of a physician.[43,44]

Antidepressants

Antidepressant medications and tranquilizers might alter nutrient status because they affect food intake or nutrient excretion. The anti-anxiety medications meprobamate, lorazepam, oxazepam, alprazolam, chlordiazepoxide (Librium), and diazepam (Valium) can cause nausea, vomiting, dry mouth, loss of appetite, diarrhea, reduced salivation, and stomach disorders.[45] The tricyclic compounds such as Elavil alter appetite and can cause weight gain or loss. These medications also increase urinary excretion and might increase losses of the B vitamins and vitamin C.[45] The side effects of monoamine oxidase (MAO) inhibitors include constipation, nausea, diarrhea, and abdominal pain and these conditions might reduce nutrient intake and excretion.[46] Diazepoxide and diazepam might alter magnesium status and increase urinary loss of calcium.

Arthritis: Treatment Medications

D-Penicillamine (Cuprimine) is used in the treatment of rheumatoid arthritis. It also is used in the treatment of heavy metal poisoning and Wilson's Disease (copper toxicity) where the medication binds to a toxic metal and carries it out of the body. In this capacity it is extremely useful. However, the medication binds other minerals that are not toxic and can contribute to mineral deficiencies.

One of the side effects of D-Penicillamine is loss of appetite, which is called anorexia. Anorexia often leads to weight loss, muscle wastage, and general malnutrition. The loss of appetite might be caused by a medication-induced deficiency of zinc. The symptoms of a zinc deficiency are diminished taste sensitivity and a reduced appetite.[47] Anyone taking D-penicillamine should consult a physician before taking a daily nutritional supplement.

Aspirin And Anti-Inflammatory Medications

Aspirin has been used as an antiseptic, a preservative, and an anti-inflammatory agent. It is predominately used in the control and alleviation of pain, headache, and the symptoms of arthritis. It is the most popular

31

medication on the market. Excessive use of aspirin can cause several nutritional side effects.

Aspirin-induced gastrointestinal bleeding is associated with increased losses of iron and iron deficiency anemia.[48] Deficiencies of folic acid, potassium, and vitamin C also are reported.[49,52] Aspirin also reduces the absorption of vitamin B_{12}.[50]

Colchicine is used in the treatment of gout, which is an inflammatory condition. Colchicine can cause increased excretion of bile, sodium, calcium, potassium, fat, and protein and can reduce the absorption of folic acid and vitamin B_{12}.[41] Adverse side effects that interfere with nutritional status include vomiting, nausea, and diarrhea.

Sulfasalazine is used for the treatment of severe inflammatory bowel disease. This medication increases the possibility of folic acid deficiency. A daily supplement of folic acid plus the inclusion of folic acid-rich foods might be necessary to prevent deficiency symptoms.

Cancer: Treatment Medications

Chemotherapy is the treatment of a disease with medications, in other words, chemical therapy. It is a common and effective treatment for many forms of cancer; however, there are many nutritional side effects to chemotherapeutic medications.

Some medications used to treat cancer cause nausea, vomiting, sore or dry mouth and throat, bloating, fullness, and other symptoms that cause aversions to food and eating. The medication 5-fluorouracil alters taste sensations and affects appetite. The results of

Table 15   **Medications and Their Nutritional Side Effects in Cancer Patients**

Name of Medication	Possible Side Effects
Mustargen, HN2, nitrogen mustard (Mechlorethamine)	Nausea, vomiting
Alkeran, L-PAM, Melphalan, (1-phenylalanine mustard)	Nausea
Cytoxan, CTX, Endoxan (Cyclophosphamide)	Nausea, vomiting, loss of appetite
Leukeran (Chlorambucil)	Nausea
Thiotepa, TSPA (triethylene-thiophosphoramide	Nausea, vomiting
Myleran (Busulfan)	Nausea
BCNU (Carmustine) CCNU (Lomustine) Methyl CCNU (Semustine)	Nausea, vomiting
5-FU (5-Fluorouracil)	Nausea, vomiting, diarrhea, mouth sores
Ara-C, Cytosar, Cytarabine (cytosine) arabinoside)	Nausea, vomiting
6-MP Purinethol (6-mercaptopurine)	Nausea
6-TG (6-thioguanine)	Nausea
Hydrea (hydroxyurea)	Nausea, vomiting
Androgens: Haoltestin, Depotestosterone, Decadurabolin, Taslac	Nausea, vomiting, liver damage

(Continued on next page)

33

Table 15	Medications and Their Nutritional Side Effects in Cancer Patients *(Cont.)*	
	Name of Medication	**Possible Side Effects**
	Dacarbazine (DTIC — Imidazole, Carboximide)	Nausea, vomiting
	Procarbazine hydrochloride (Methyl hydrazine, Ibenzmethyzin, Matulane)	Nause, vomiting
	Cisplatin (Platinol, Cis-platinum, DDP)	Nausea, vomiting

these conditions are loss of appetite, malnutrition, tissue wastage, and weight loss.[53,54] *(Table 15)*

Other chemotherapeutic medications damage the lining of the intestinal tract or cause diarrhea, which reduces nutrient absorption and increases the excretion of nutrients.

Some medications used to treat cancer interfere with the use of nutrients in cells. For example, methotrexate is a medication used for the treatment of cancer and psoriasis. It exerts its therapeutic effect by altering folic acid metabolism. Folic acid is important in normal cell and tissue growth. Methotrexate blocks the enzyme necessary for the conversion of dietary folic acid to its biologically active form and cells cannot divide or grow. Since cancer cells divide more rapidly than normal cells, a medication-induced folic acid deficiency exerts a greater effect on these diseased cells. Methotrexate affects all folic acid-dependent reactions in the body, however, including healthy cells. Red blood cells do not divide properly and megaloblastic anemia is common in patients taking methotrexate.

People taking methotrexate should not self-medicate with folic acid supplements without the prior consent of a physician. Large doses of the vitamin could alter the effectiveness of the medication therapy.[55]

Another medication-nutrient interaction common in cancer therapy is a thiamin deficiency caused by 5-fluorouracil.[56] A loss of fluids, electrolytes, and proteins caused by vomiting and diarrhea can reduce nutrient intake and contribute to malnutrition.

Oral Contraceptives

Oral contraceptives affect food intake and nutritional status in several ways. They have been reported to do the following:

- Increase appetite and encourage weight gain
- Impair glucose tolerance
- Increase blood levels of cholesterol and triglycerides
- Reduce absorption of folic acid
- Promote water retention (edema)

Oral contraceptives are associated with several nutrient deficiencies. Some women who take oral contraceptives exhibit hight blood levels of vitamin A and low blood levels of vitamin E, vitamin C, vitamin B_6, folic acid, vitamin B_1 (thiamin), vitamin B_2 (riboflavin), vitamin B_{12}, zinc, iron, and total iron binding capacity, which is another sign of compromised iron status.[42,57,60] Blood levels of copper can be high in these women.[62]

Some individuals are more sensitive to medication-nutrient interactions than other individuals. Nutrient deficiencies also are dependent on the particular oral contraceptive used, the length of time it is used, and the nutritional status and age of the woman prior to the use of the product.

Vitamin B_6 is of particular interest because of its role in mood and behavior. (Appendix A) When daily intake is increased from the RDA of 2 mg to 20 to 40 mg daily, the depression associated with birth control pills might be alleviated.[63]

Heart Disease: Medications To Lower Cholesterol

Some medications, such as cholestyramine, clofibrate, colestipol, and neomycin (See page 29 for information on neomycin), are used in the treatment of heart disease because they bind cholesterol and bile acids in the intestines and prevent their reabsorption. This reduces circulating blood levels of cholesterol. Elevated blood cholesterol levels are associated with an increased risk for heart disease.

These medications also bind other fat-soluble substances such as the fat-soluble vitamins and essential fatty acids, which might cause vitamin K deficiency, vitamin D deficiency, and related bone disorders.[64,65] Other symptoms of fat-soluble vitamin deficiencies include night blindness, the destruction of red blood cells (anemia), and hemorrhage.

Cholestyramine (Questran) is a cholesterol-lowering medication given to patients with high blood cholesterol levels. It can cause steatorrhea (fatty stools) and malabsorption of the fat-soluble vitamins A, D, E, and K.[66] Iron, carotene, calcium, vitamin B_{12}, and folic acid deficiencies also might

36

occur.[67,68] Bone disorders and anemia might result. Cholestyramine increases urinary excretion of calcium, increases blood levels of triglycerides, and reduces body stores of iron when taken over a long period of time or at high doses.

Clofibrate binds cholesterol and bile acids in the intestines and reduces their reabsorption; therefore, blood cholesterol levels are reduced. Besides the potential for increased excretion of the fat-soluble vitamins, this medication changes the taste sensation, which might reduce a person's desire to eat.

Colestipol is another medication used in the treatment of heart disease. Deficiencies of the fat-soluble vitamins A, D, and E and folic acid are possible when this medication is taken.[57] Vitamin K supplementation is required only in the presence of poor blood clotting and prolonged bleeding times. The effectiveness of colestipol is increased when it is combined with the B vitamin nicotinic acid (niacin).[69]

Hyperactivity: Treatment Medications

Dextroamphetamine (Dexadrine) and a similar compound methylphenidate (Ritalin) are used to control behavioral problems in hyperactive children. These stimulants calm, rather than excite, hyperactive patients. Growth retardation has been noted in hyperactive children who are on long-term medication therapy.[70] This side effect might be a result of reduced food intake associated with medication-induced suppression of appetite.

Hypertension: Treatment Medications

The diurétic medications (water pills) used in the treatment of hypertension and congestive heart failure include the thiazides, furosemide, and ethacrynic acid. These medications increase the urinary loss of potassium and other minerals, as well as water. Most physicians are aware of the potential loss of potassium with the use of diuretics and recommend that people take a potassium supplement. If a potassium deficiency were allowed to progress, a person might experience bone fragility, paralysis, sterility, muscle weakness, nerve disorders, irregular heart beat (arrhythmias), and kidney damage.[71]

People taking potassium-depleting diuretics should include potassium-rich foods in the diet daily. (Appendix C)

Not everyone who takes a diuretic needs to be concerned about potassium depletion. Some diuretics, such as spironolactone, are not associated with a deficiency of the mineral.

Consult a physician to see if a diuretic requires supplementation with potassium before self-medicating.

Other medications that deplete the body of potassium include:

- L-DOPA
- Senna
- Gentamicin
- Amphotericin B
- Bisacodyl
- Salicylates
- Phenolphthalein
- Corticosteroids

Magnesium is another mineral that can be depleted with the use of thiazides. Magnesium functions in energy production, the manufacture of fat and protein, the removal of toxic compounds such as urea and ammonia, muscle relaxation, nerve transmission, the prevention of tooth decay, the transportation of nutrients into the cells, and bone formation and maintenance. A deficiency of this mineral affects the heart, nerves, and kidneys. Low magnesium in the body might cause arrhythmias (irregular heart beat), heart failure, atherosclerosis, destruction of the heart muscle, and convulsions.[72] In some cases, magnesium supplements eliminate the incidence of heart attack in people prone to cardiovascular disease.[73,74]

The American diet is already low in magnesium.[74] This potential nutritional risk is aggravated by the addition of magnesium-depleting medications that might cause conditions such as heart and vascular diseases. A diet high in magnesium or magnesium supplementation might reduce the risk for heart and vascular disease and is recommended for persons taking thiazide diuretics. *(Table 16)*

Mineral deficiencies of calcium, iodine, and zinc are associated with the use of furosemide and ethacrynic acid.[68]

Prolonged use of diuretics could place a person at risk for deficiencies of the water-soluble vitamins, which are vitamin C and the B vitamins. The antihypertensive medication hydrazine (Apresoline) interferes with vitamin B_6 metabolism and causes deficiency symptoms that include behavioral disorders (Appendix A), sleep irregularities, and convulsions.[75] A vitamin supplement that provides

Table 16	Medications That Affect Magnesium Status
	Medication
Alcohol	Phenobarbital
Amphotericin B	Phenytoin
Capreomycin	Tetracyclines
Carbenicillin	Thiazides
Cisplatin	Tobramicin
Cyclocerine	Viomycin
Digitalis glycosides	Mercurial diuretics
Ethracrynic acid	— chlormerodrin
Furosemide	— meralluride
Gentamicin	— mercaptomerin
Lithium	— mercurophylline
	— mersalyl

approximately 100% of the Recommended Dietary Allowance (RDA) for the nine B vitamins and vitamin C might prevent potential deficiencies.

Laxatives

Laxatives impair the absorption of nutrients from the intestines. The laxatives phenolphthalein (Alophen, Ex-lax, Feen-a-mint), senna (Senokot), and bisacodyl (Dulcolax) increase the activity of the intestines and alter the intestinal lining.[76] As a result, several nutrients, such as calcium, potassium, and vitamin D, are excreted rather than absorbed.

Another laxative, mineral oil, binds the fat-soluble nutrients, the essential fatty acids, and the fat-soluble vitamins A, D, E, and K. Mineral oil is not absorbed, so both the oil and the essential nutrients

Table 17	Nutritional Effects of Laxative Use	
	Type of Laxative	Nutritional Consequences
	Bisacodyl, Phenol Phthalein, Senna	Hypokalemia, and potassium deficiency
	Bisacodyl, Phenol-phthalein, Senna Mineral Oil	Malabsorption syndromes
	Phenolphthalein	Protein-losing enteropathy

are excreted.[77-79] As little as 4 teaspoons of this laxative used daily can produce deficiency symptoms of the fat-soluble vitamins.

Symptoms of vitamin A deficiency include poor vision at night (night blindness), reduced resistance to infection, skin problems such as dermatitis, and abnormal bone and tooth development. Inadequate intake of vitamin D can result in bone problems such as osteomalacia. A deficiency of vitamin K causes hemorrhage. The skin, blood, and nerves are affected by a vitamin E deficiency. Without essential fats, the skin becomes rough, dry, and scaly.

A high-fiber, low-fat diet that provides at least 8 glasses of water daily and is combined with a personalized exercise program can aid in the relief of constipation without the side effects of chronic laxative use.

Steroids

Steroids are a group of medications that are used to increase muscle mass in athletes, and include oral contraceptives and estrogen.

Estrogen use can cause abdominal cramping, loss of appetite, diarrhea, and nausea. These side effects can reduce food and nutrient intake or increase nutrient losses. Salt and fluid retention and weight gain also are possible.

Tuberculosis: Treatment Medications

Isoniazide (INH) is used in the long-term treatment of tuberculosis. This medication can cause dry mouth, loss of appetite, nausea, stomach distress, and vomiting. The potential nutritional side effects include a vitamin B_6 deficiency. INH binds to the vitamin and the two are excreted in the urine. When other antituberulosis medications, such as cycloserine and pyrazinamide, are taken with INH, anemia can develop. When a person is taking one or more of these medications, daily supplementation with 50mg of vitamin B_6 might protect against a deficiency.[53]

Weight Control Pills

A medication used in weight loss pills is phenylpropanolamine (PPA). This substance is ineffective in permanent weight loss; the weight gain exceeds weight loss. The average weekly weight loss is less than half a pound. In addition, more than 10,000 cases of toxic effects attributed to phenylpropanolamine have been reported to FDA's Poison Control Center; 1000 of these cases were emergency room visits. Its side effects include the following:

- increased blood pressure
- restlessness
- irritability
- anxiety
- insomnia
- headaches

The side effects related to anxiety and pain can reduce a person's desire for food and interfere with nutrient intake and absorption.

Consult Tables 18 and 19 for the nutritional effects of other medications and general dietary recommendations.

Table 18　Drug-Nutrient Interactions

Medication	Use	Effect on Nutritional Status
Alcohol	Toxic effect on intestinal lining, altered secretion of digestive enzymes	Reduced absorption of vitamin B_1, folic acid, vitamin B_2; increased excretion of magnesium and zinc; reduced blood levels of vitamin B_{12}.
Amitriptyline Imipramine Lithium carbonate	Antidepressant	Weight gain; altered blood glucose; increased blood levels of magnesium; increased excretion of calcium.
Amphotericin B	Antifungal	Increased urinary excretion of potassium and nitrogen; reduced blood levels of magnesium and potassium.
Antihistamines	Nasal Congstion	Increases appetite.
Barbiturates	Anticonvulsant	Increased need for folic acid and vitamin D; reduced absorption of vitamin B_1; increased excretion of vitamin C.
Biouanides Metformin, Phenformin	Diabetes	Reduces absorption of vitamin B_{12}
Chloramphenicol	Antimicrobial	Increased need for vitamin B_2, vitamin B_6, and vitamin B_{12}.
Chlorpromazine	Tranquilizer	Increased appetite and body weight.
Colchicine	Anti-inflammatory	Reduces absorption of carotene, sodium, potassium, vitamin B_{12}, lactose.
Colocynth	Cathartic	Reduces transit time and absorption of nutrients.

(Continued on next page)

44

Table 18   Drug-Nutrient Interactions *(Cont.)*

Medication	Use	Effect on Nutritional Status
Corticosteroids		Reduced absorption of calcium and phosphorus; increased urinary excretion of vitamin C, calcium, potassium, zinc, and nitrogen; reduced blood levels of zinc; increased blood levels of glucose, triglycerides, and cholesterol; increased need for vitamin B_6, vitamin C, folic acid, and vitamin D; impaired bone formation; reduced wound healing.
Coumarin	Anticoagulant	Antagonist to vitamin K.
Cycloserine	Antitubercular	Reduced protein synthesis; reduced absorption of calcium and magnesium; reduced blood levels of folic acid, vitamin B_{12}, and vitamin B_6.
Dextroam-phetamine	Appetite suppressant	Weight loss, reduced growth in children.
Indomethacin	Analgesic	Reduced blood level of vitamin C; reduced absorption of amino acids; anemia.
Insulin	Diabetes	Increases appetite.
Glutethimide	Sedative-hynotic	Increased need for vitamin D.
Griseofulvin	Antifungal	Alters taste sensitivity.
Hydralazine	Hypotensive	Increased excretion of vitamin B_6.
Isotretinoin (a synthetic derivative of vitamin A)	Acne	Avoid supplementation with vitamin A (41).

(Continued on next page)

45

Table 18   Drug-Nutrient Interactions *(Cont.)*

Medication	Use	Effect on Nutritional Status
Jalap	Cathartic	Reduces transit time and absorption of nutrients.
Kaon-Cl	Potassium	Reduces absorption of vitamin B_{12}.
K-Tab	Potassium	Reduces absorption of vitamin B_{12}.
Klotrix	Potassium	Reduces absorption of vitamin B_{12}.
Lithium carbonate	Tranquilizer	Increases appetite and body weight.
Methylphenidate	Appetite suppressant	Weight loss and reduced growth in children.
Micro-K	Potassium	Reduces absorption of vitamin B_{12}.
Paraaminosali-cyclic acid	Antitubercular	Reduced absorption of vitamin B_{12}, iron, folic acid, and fat.
Penicillins	Antimicrobial	Reduced blood levels of potassium.
Phenobarbital Phenytoin Primidone	Anticonvulsant	Impaired vitamin D metabolism; increased excretion of vitamin D; reduced blood levels of folic acid, vitamin B_{12}, and vitamin B_6; anemia.
Podophyllin	Cathartic	Reduces transit time and absorption of nutrients.
Propranolol	Cardiac	Reduced glucose tolerance.
Slow-K	Potassium	Reduces absorption of vitamin B_{12}.

(Continued on next page)

Table 18   Drug-Nutrient Interactions *(Cont.)*

Medication	Use	Effect on Nutritional Status
Sodium nitro-prusside	Hypotensive	Increased urinary excretion of vitamin B_{12}; reduced blood level of vitamin B_{12}.
Sulfasalazine	Ulcerative Colitis	Reduces absorption of folic acid and reduces intestinal transit time.
Thiazides	Diuretics	Increased urinary excretion of potassium, magnesium, zinc, and vitamin B_2.
Viomycin	Antimicrobial	Reduced blood levels of potassium and calcium; alkalosis.

Table 19 **Drug-Nutrient Interactions and Dietary Recommendations**

Drug	Effects on Nutritional Status	Dietary Recommendations
Antacids	Bloating, constipation, nausea. Reduces phosphate, reduces vitamin A, loss of appetite.	Take between meals. Increase intake of vitamin. A, iron, and folic acid.
Bisacodyl (laxative)	Diarrhea, nausea, fluid loss. Reduces absorption of glucose. Hypokalemia (loss of potassium).	Take on empty stomach. with water. Increase water intake.
Cholestyramine (Lipid lowering)	Belching, bloating, constipation, diarrhea flatulence, stearorrhea.	Increase intake of fat-soluble vitamins, carotene, iron, B_{12}, and calcium. High fiber diet if constipated.
Colchicine (antigout)	Diarrhea, nausea, vomiting. Reduces absorption or increases excretion of sodium potassium, fat, carotene B_{12}, folic acid, calcium.	Take with water and food. Avoid alcohol. Increase fluid intake. Supplement or increase dietary intake of high risk nutrients.
Furosemide (Diuretic)	Constipation, diarrhea nausea, or vomiting. Increased excretion of potassium, calcium, magnesium, sodium, water. Dry mouth, loss of appetite.	Take single dose early in morning.
Hydralzine (antihyper-tensive)	Diarrhea, constipation, nausea. Reduces B_6, loss of appetite, and sodium retention.	Take with food. Maintain ideal weight. Vitamin B_6 supplementation. Sodium restriction.

(Continued on next page)

48

Table 19   Drug-Nutrient Interactions and Dietary Recommendations (Cont.)

Drug	Effects on Nutritional Status	Dietary Recommendations
Isoniazid (anti-tubercular)	Stomach distress nausea, vomiting. Reduced B_6. Dry mouth. Loss of appetite.	Take on empty stomach. Avoid alcohol. Vitamin B_6 supplementation.
Methotrexate (cancer)	Diarrhea, GI bleeding, nausea or vomiting. Reduces folic acid. Poor absorption of B_{12} Loss of appetite, sore mouth and throat, altered taste.	Increase water intake. Avoid alcohol.
Mineral Oil (laxative)	Flatulence, nausea, vomiting. Reduces absorption of vitamins A, D, E, K. Loss of appetite and weight loss. Hypokalemia (Low potassium).	Take 2 hours before a meal. Increase fat-soluble vitamin intake.
Penicillamine (Antiarthritic)	Diarrhea, nausea vomiting. Reduces copper, zinc, and iron. Altered taste taste and loss of appetite.	Take with water. Take on empty stomach. B_6 and trace mineral supplementation.
Phenolphthalein (laxative)	Reduced absorption of vitamin D, calcium, and other minerals. Hypokalemia (low potassium).	Take on empty stomach. Chew well.
Phenylbutazone (antiin-flammatory)	Constipation, diarrhea heartburn, fluid retention, and weight gain.	Take with food. Avoid alcohol.

(Continued on next page)

49

Table 19   Drug-Nutrient Interactions and Dietary Recommendations (Cont.)

Drug	Effects on Nutritional Status	Dietary Recommendations
Steroids	Bloating, indigestion, nausea. Fluid and sodium retention. Reduced absorption of vitamin D. Osteomalacia.	Take with food or low-sodium snack. Sodium-restricted diet. Increase potassium.
Steroids (Anabolic)	Nausea, vomiting, fluid retention, edema, and weight gain.	
Sulfasalazine (Antiinflammatory)	Diarrhea, stomach distress, nausea, vomiting. Reduces absorption of folic acid. Loss of appetite.	Take with water. Increase water intake. Increase folic acid-rich foods.

4
How Food Affects the Action of Medications

Food could increase a medication's effect, decrease its effect, or prevent its usefulness. Eating certain foods while taking some medications might be dangerous. Food can increase or decrease the absorption or excretion of a medication or interfere with its metabolic effects. It is because of these interactions that a physician will recommend that some medications be taken before, during, or between meals.

Food can reduce the absorption of a medication and reduce the medication's effectiveness. An example is the interaction between tetracycline and dairy products. The calcium in cheese, milk, and yogurt forms insoluble complexes with tetracycline in the intestines and inhibits its absorption. There is no need to eliminate these foods from the diet; consume them at times other than when the medication is taken.

Several nutrients interact with tetracycline. Vitamin A in doses of 50,000 IU in combination with tetracycline can cause intracranial pressure (severe headaches).[80] Calcium, magnesium, zinc, and iron form insoluble complexes with the antibiotic and reduce its absorption. For instance, when iron is taken for anemia at the same time that tetracycline is taken for an infection, the effects of both are lost.

This does not mean that these nutrients and these foods should be avoided when taking tetracycline, only that they should be taken at different times than the medication.[81]

The rate of absorption of many antibiotic medications, such as sulfanilamide, erythromycin, and metronidazole, is reduced when taken with food. In contrast, other anti-infective medications, such as griseofulvin and sulfamethoxydiazine have increased absorption when taken with food.[82]

Anyone suffering from depression or high blood pressure who is taking a monoamine oxidase (MAO) inhibitor such as isocarboxazid (Marplan), phenelzine (Nardil), and tranylcypromine (Parnate) should avoid all aged or fermented foods. These include pickled herring, fermented sausages (salami and pepperoni), sharp or aged cheese, yogurt, sour cream, beef and chicken livers, canned figs, bananas, avocados, soy sauce, meat tenderizers, yeast, beer, Chianti wine, sherry, and other wines in large amounts. MAO inhibitors also might react with substances in cola beverages, coffee, and chocolate. The medication reacts with substances in these foods and might produce high blood pressure, headaches, and brain hemorrhage.

Excessive consumption of vitamin K-rich foods, such as liver and dark green leafy vegetables, can interfere with anticoagulant therapy. Vitamin K promotes blood clotting, which is in opposition to the effects of Coumarin and other anticoagulants. Again, these food need not be eliminated, but moderation should be exercised in their use.

Table 20	The Effects of Food on Absorption and Action of Medications	
Food	**Drug**	**Action**
Coffee/tea	Neuroleptic agents	Reduces drug absorption
	Theophylline	Increases drug side effects
Citrus	Quinidine	Increases blood levels of drug
Fiber (bran, Pectin)	Digoxin	Reduces drug absorption
Food/meals	Chlorothiazide	Increases drug absorption
	Propranolol	Increases drug absorption
	Nitrofurantoin	Increases drug effectiveness
	Cimetidine	Delays drug absorption
	Aspirin	Reduces drug absorption
	Tetracycline	Reduces drug absorption
High-fat foods	Griseofulvin	Increases drug absorption
High-protein foods	Levodopa, methyldopa	Reduces drug absorption
Licorice	Antihypertensive drugs	Induces hypokalemia and sodium retention
Milk	Tetracycline	Reduces drug absorption

(Continued on next page)

Table 20	The Effects of Food on Absorption and Action of Medications *(Cont.)*	
Food	**Drug**	**Action**
Meal with Milk	Methotrexate	Reduces drug absorption
Salty foods	Lithium	Reduces drug effectiveness
Vegetables (dark green)	Warfarin	Reduces drug effectiveness

To Avoid Adverse Medication or Prescription Drug-Nutrient Interactions:

1. Read labels on non-prescription medications. Check for any dietary guidelines that should be followed while taking the medication.
2. Follow the orders of a physician about when to take a medication and what foods or beverages to avoid.
3. Do not hesitate to ask how medications might react with the foods.
4. Eat a nutritionally balanced diet that includes a variety of foods.
5. If a person has been on a medication, whether it is a prescription drug or a non-prescription drug, for a long time and has noticed signs or symptoms that are not related to the disease or side effects of the medication, then a medication-induced nutrient deficiency is possible. These signs and symptoms should be discussed with a physician.
6. For added nutritional protection, vitamin-mineral formulas have been developed to counteract medication-induced malnutrition. (Appendix D) *(Table 20, page 53, 54)*

Appendix A: Vitamin B$_6$ and Temperament

Behavioral changes are a common side effect of several prescription and non-prescription medications. These medications might affect mood and personality because of their effect on how vitamin B$_6$ is used in the body.

Vitamin B$_6$ is an essential component in the body's production of several neurotransmitters and hormones. These substances regulate behavior and numerous body processes. For example, serotonin is a principal neurotransmitter found in the brain. It is produced from the amino acid tryptophan in the presence of vitamin B$_6$. Serotonin regulates biological and psychological functions including sleep, emotions, and mood. Low levels of serotonin are associated with depression, insomnia, and seizures.[83,85] Medications that raise the level of serotonin can affect behavior.

The brain depends on what is eaten to regulate the production of serotonin. The level of serotonin is regulated by the amount of tryptophan and vitamin B$_6$ in the diet; chronically low intake of either or both can result in reduced production of serotonin and might cause mood disorders.[86] Medications such as steroid hormones, oral contraceptives, and antituberculous medications (INH) interfere with vitamin B$_6$ metabolism and suppress the synthesis of serotonin. The mood swings and depression that often accompany these medications are reduced or eliminated when vitamin B$_6$ supplements are taken.

A physician should be consulted before a supplement is taken, since in some cases vitamin B$_6$ can inhibit the effectiveness of a medication. For instance, vitamin B_6 supplementation is not indicated when L-DOPA is used in the treatment of Parkinson's disease.[87]

Vitamin B_6 supplementation is recommended when the following medications are used:

- Apresoline
- Donnatal
- Deltasone
- Medrol
- Oral Contraceptives
- Premarin
- Serapes

Appendix B: Dietary Sources of Vitamins and Minerals

Nutrient	Dietary Source
Vitamin A	Dark green and orange vegetables and fruits (ie., carrots, apricots, spinach), liver.
Vitamin D	Fortified milk, fish oils.
Vitamin E	Vegetable oils, whole grain breads and cereals, dark green leafy vegetables.
Vitamin K	Dark green leafy vegetables.
Vitamin B_1	Pork, beef, organ meats, whole grain cereals and breads, nuts, legumes.
Vitamin B_2	Milk, cheese, yogurt, mushrooms, broccoli, avocados.
Niacin	Organ meats, peanuts, meat, poultry, fish, legumes, milk
Vitamin B_6	Meat, organ meats, poultry, fish, soybeans, dried beans.

Folic Acid*	Dark green vegetables, dried beans, orange juice, cantaloupe, green peas, sweet potatoes.
Vitamin B_{12}	Meat, poultry, fish, clams, oysters, milk, cheese, fermented soybean products.
Biotin	Liver, organ meats, molasses, milk.
Pantothenic Acid	Meat, fish, chicken, cheese, whole grain cereals and breads, avocados, green peas, dried beans, nuts, dates.
Vitamin C*	Fresh fruits and vegetables.
Calcium	Milk, yogurt, cheese, dark green leafy vegetables.
Chromium	Whole grain breads and cereals, meats.
Copper	Whole grain breads and cereals, shellfish, nuts, organ meats, dried beans and peas, dark green leafy vegetables.
Iron	Meat, liver, dried fruits, legumes, dark green leafy vegetables, prune juice, oysters, strawberries, watermelon, broccoli.
Magnesium	Nuts, legumes, whole grain breads and cereals, soybeans, seafood, dark green leafy vegetables.
Manganese	Liver, lettuce, spinach, whole grain cereals and breads, dried beans and peas, nuts.
Potassium	Meat, milk, fruits, potatoes, bananas, orange juice, dried fruits.
Selenium	Meats, poultry, seafood. Content in grains and vegetables will vary depending on selenium content of soil in which they are grown.

| Zinc | Oysters, milk, meat, whole grain cereals and breads. |

*Losses occur if food is stored, cooked too long, reheated, or if water used in cooking is discarded.

Appendix C: Symptoms Associated With Vitamin and Mineral Deficiencies

Nutrient	Deficiency Symptom
Vitamin A	Skin disorders, poor night vision, reduced resistance to infection, poor bone and tooth development.
Vitamin D	Rickets or osteomalacia.
Vitamin E	Anemia, reproductive system damage.
Vitamin K	Hemorrhage.
Vitamin B_1	Fatigue, anorexia, weight loss, gastrointestinal problems, weakness, nausea, numbness and tingling in the hands and feet, memory loss, reduced attention span, irritability, confusion.
Vitamin B_2	Cracks at the corners of the mouth, inflammation of the mouth, reddening of the eyes, burning and itching of the eyes, dermatitis, depression.
Niacin	Dermatitis, diarrhea, irritability, headache, insomnia, memory loss.
Vitamin B_6	Weakness, mental confusion, irritability, nervousness, insomnia, poor coordination, anemia, dermatitis.
Folic Acid	Anemia, irritability, weakness, weight loss, apathy, headache, forgetfulness, gastrointestinal problems, diarrhea.

Vitamin B$_{12}$	Anemia, anorexia, gastrointestinal problems, fatigue, dizziness, numbness and tingling, moodiness.
Vitamin C	Anemia, joint tenderness and swelling, poor wound healing, weakness, bleeding gums, bruising.
Calcium	Osteoporosis.
Chromium	Glucose insensitivity resembling diabetes.
Copper	Low white blood cell count, poor collagen formation, bone deterioration, anemia.
Iron	Anemia, lethargy, poor concentration, paleness, headaches.
Magnesium	Lethargy, weakness, confusion, personality changes, muscle tremors, anorexia, nausea, lack of coordination, gastrointestinal problems, heart disease and arrhythmia.
Manganese	No established deficiency symptoms in humans.
Potassium	Impaired growth, bone weakness, sterility, muscle weakness, reduced heart rate.
Selenium	Structural damage to the heart.
Zinc	Changes in hair and nails, sterility, skin disorders, lethargy, anemia, poor wound healing, loss of taste and smell.

Appendix D: Guidelines For Supplementation When Taking Medications

Medications might affect a person's nutritional state by one of a number of means, including reduced food intake or absorption of nutrients; altered distribution, storage, or use of a nutrient in the body; increased need for a nutrient; and increased excretion of a vitamin or mineral. This interference may be undesirable and, in some cases, might result in marginal to obvious nutrient deficiencies.[6] The nutritional side effects of some medications might be prevented or improved by proper diet and supplementation.

Research in the area of medication-nutrient interactions is limited; few specialists exist and many medication categories have not been investigated. Although information is available on the effects of certain foods on medication absorption and excretion and how the medication is used in the body, it is less clear to what degree medications alter nutrient availabililty and excretion. Some medications might alter a single nutrient, while other medications might alter several nutrients. When multiple nutrients are invloved, a balanced nutritional supplement that avoids possible nutrient-medication and nutrient-nutrient interactions might be a consideration.

A number of companies are introducing vitamin and mineral formulas to compensate for potential nutrient inadequacies that might be associated with the ingestion of certain medications. A review of the literature by members of Health Media's Editorial Board has produced a list of nutrients that should be considered when a person evaluates nutritional supplement formulas designed for certain medications and medication categories. If you are currently taking a vitamin-mineral supplement, check the formula for the nutrients listed opposite the generic or brand name of your medication.

If you are taking medications and are considering a nutritional supplement, be sure to discuss this issue with your pharmacist. The information contained in this book is provided only as an introduction to the subject of medication-induced malnutrition and should be used in conjunction with the advice of a pharmacist or physician.

These nutrients: **Might decrease the risk of nutrient imbalance associated with the following medications:**

Nutrients	Medications
Vitamin B_1	Aldactazide
Vitamin B_2	Aldoril
Niacinamide	Dyazide
Vitamin B_6	Enduron
Vitamin B_{12}	Esidrex
Folic acid	Hygroton
Magnesium	Hydrodiuril
Zinc	Hydrochlorothiazide
Chromium	Hydropres
Manganese	Inderide
Potassium	Moduretic
Copper	
Calcium	

These nutrients: **Might decrease the risk of nutrient imbalance associated with the following medications:**

Nutrients	Medications
Calcium	Lanoxin
Magnesium	Lasix

These nutrients: Might decrease the risk of nutrient imbalance associated with the following medications:

Nutrients	Medications
Vitamin B_1	Achromycin V
Vitamin B_2	Aldomet
Niacinamide	Bactrim
Pantothenic acid	Bactrim DS
Vitamin B_6	Mellaril
Vitamin B_{12}	Oral Contraceptives
Folic acid	Septra
Vitamin C	Stelazine
Zinc	Sumycin
Copper	Tetracycline
	Thorazine
	Triavil
	Vibramycin
	Vibra Tabs

These nutrients: Might decrease the risk of nutrient imbalance associated with the following medications:

Nutrients	Medications
Calcium	Dilantin
Magnesium	Phenobarbital
Vitamin D	
Vitamin B_6	
Folic acid	
Vitamin B_{12}	
Vitamin B_1	
Vitamin B_2	
Niacinamide	

These nutrients: **Might decrease the risk of nutrient imbalance associated with the following medications:**

Nutrients

Vitamin C
Folic acid
Iron
Vitamin E
Vitamin K

Medications

Aspirin and aspirin containing medications, such as Empirin Codine, Darvon, Synalgos DC, and Percodan

References

1. Hall R: Psychiatric and physiological reactions produced by Over the Counter drugs. *J Psychedelic Drugs* 1978;10:423-426.
2. Garrison R, Somer E: *The Nutrition Desk Reference.* New Canaan, Conn., Keats Publishing Co, 1985, p 210.
3. *Facts and Comparisons: Drug Information.* St. Louis, J.B. Lippencott Co, 1985, p 189.
4. Hayes J, Borzelleca J: Nutrient interaction with drugs and other xenobiotics. *J Am Diet A* 1985; 85:335-339.
5. Bren M: Erythrocyte as a biopsy tissue in the functional evaluation of thiamine status. *JAMA* 1964; 187:762.
6. Garrison R, Somer E: *The Nutrition Desk Reference.* New Canaan, Conn., Keats Publishing Co, 1985, pp 210-212.
7. Roe D: *Drug-Induced Nutritional Deficiencies.* Westport, Conn., The AVI Publishing Co, 1983, p 39.
8. Garrison R, Somer E: *The Nutrition Desk Reference.* New Canaan, Conn., Keats Publishing Co, 1985, p 212.
9. Ibid, p 48.
10. Ibid, p 217.
11. Roe D: *Drug-Induced Nutritional Deficiencies.* Westport, Conn., The AVI Publishing Co, 1983, pp 253-254.
12. Roe D: Drug-food and drug-nutrient interactions. *J Env P Tox* 1985; 5:115-135.
13. *Statistical Abstracts of the United States.* US Dept of Commerce, Bureau of the Census, Washington DC, 1980.
14. Chien C, Townsend E, Townsend A: Substance use and abuse among the community elderly: The medical aspect. *Addict Dis* 1978; 3:357-372.
15. Guttman P: Patterns of legal drug use by older Americans. *Addict Dis.* 1978; 3:337-356.
16. Gibson R, Mueller M, Fisher C: Age differences in healthcare spending. Fiscal Year 1976. *Soc Sec Bull* 1977; 40:314.
17. Roe D: *Drugs and Nutrition in the Geriatric Patient.* New York, Churchill Livingstone, 1984, p 9.
18. Ibid, p 9.
19. Garrison R, Somer E: *The Nutrition Desk Reference.* New Canaan, Conn., Keats Publishing Co, 1985, p 220.
20. Tomasula P, Keter R, Iber F: Impairment of thiamin absorption in alcoholism. *Am J Clin Nutr* 1968; 21:1340.
21. Halsted C, Robles E, Mezey E: Intestinal malabsorption in folate deficient alcoholics. *Gastroenterology* 1973; 64:526.
22. Garrison R, Somer E: *The Nutrition Desk Reference.* New Canaan, Conn., Keats Publishing Co, 1985, p 210-211.

23. Spencer H, Norris C, Coffey F, et al: Effect of small amounts of antacids on calcium, phosphorus and flouride metabolism in man. *Gastroenterology* 1975; 68:990.

24. Lotz M, Zisman E, Bartter F: Evidence for a phosphorusdepletion syndrome in man. *N Engl J Med* 1968; 278:409.

25. Bloom W, Flinchum D: Osteomalacia with pseudofractures caused by the ingestion of aluminum hydroxide. *JAMA* 1960; 174:1327.

26. Mahan L, Krause M: *Food, Nutrition, and Diet Therapy* ed 7. Philadelphia, WB Saunders Co., 1984, p 431.

27. Ibid, p 412-414.

28. Benn A, Swan C, Cooke W, et al: Effect of intraluminal pH on the absorption of pterylmonoglutamic acid. *Br Med J* 1971; 1:148.

29. McGuigan J: A consideration of the adverse effects of cimetidine. *Gastroenterology* 1980; 80:181.

30. Diet-Drug interactions. *Dairy Council Digest* 1977; 48:7-11.

31. Roe D: *Drug-Induced Nutritional Deficiencies.* Westport, Conn., The AVI Publishing Co, 1983, p 27.

32. Ibid, p 44.

33. Mahan L, Krause M: *Food, Nutrition, and Diet Therapy.* Philadelphia, WB Saunders Co, 1984, pp 419-420.

34. Roe D: *Drug-Induced Nutritional Deficiencies.* Westport, Conn., The AVI Publishing Co, 1983, pp 130-133.

35. Christakis G, Christakis P: Drug-interactions nutrients, vitamins, foods. *Vitamin Communications,* Hoffmann-La Roche Inc. Nutley, New Jersey, 07110

36. Roe D: *Drugs and Nutrition in the Geriatric Patient.* New York, Churchill Livingston, 1984, pp 111-112.

37. Garrison R, Somer E: *The Nutrition Desk Reference.* New Canaan, Conn., Keats Publishing Co, 1985, p 211.

38. Roe D: *Drug-Induced Nutritional Deficiencies.* Westport, Conn., The AVI Publishing Co, 1983, pp 54,125-126,137.

39. Roe D: *Drug-Nutrient Interactions,* prepared for Hoffmann-LaRoche, Inc.

40. Roe D: *Drug-Induced Nutritional Deficiencies.* Westport, Conn., The AVI Publishing Co, 1983, p 191.

41. Mahan L, Krause M: *Food, Nutrition, and Diet Therapy.* Philadelphia, WB Saunders Co, 1984, p 414.

42. Ibid, p 418.

43. Relieving the analgesic headache. Time 110 (August 1, 1977). *The Weekly News Magazine;* copyright *Time Inc.* 1977.

44. Baum C, Selhub J, Rosenberg I: Antifolate actions of sulfasalazine on intact lymphocytes. *J Lab Clin Med* 1981; 97:779

45. *Facts and Comparisons: Drug Information.* St. Louis, J.B. Lippencott Co.,1985, pp 260-264.

46. Ibid, p 261C.
47. Garrison R, Somer E: *The Nutrition Desk Reference.* New Canaan, Conn., Keats Publishing Co, 1985, pp 57-78.
48. Roe D: *Drug-Induced Nutritional Deficiencies.* Westport, Conn., The AVI Publishing Co, 1983, pp 45,121.
49. Ibid, p 16.
50. Mahan L, Krause M: *Food, Nutrition, and Diet Therapy* ed 7. Philadelphia, WB Saunders Co, 1984, p 409.
51. Ibid, p 414.
52. Roe D: *Drug-Induced Nutritional Deficiencies.* Westport, Conn., The AVI Publishing Co, 1983, pp 151-152.
53. Mahan L, Krause M: *Food, Nutrition, and Diet Therapy* ed 7. Philadelphia, WB Saunders Co, 1984, p 413.
54. Ibid, pp 744-746.
55. Roe D: *Drug-Induced Nutritional Deficiencies.* Westport, Conn., The AVI Publishing Co, 1983, 12,16,96.
56. Ibid, p 20.
57. Garrison R, Somer E: *The Nutrition Desk Reference.* New Canaan, Conn., Keats Publishing Co, 1985, pp 215-218.
58. Mahan L, Krause M: *Food, Nutrition, and Diet Therapy* ed 7. Philadelphia, WB Saunders Co, 1984, pp 418-419.
59. Roe D: *Drug-Induced Nutritional Deficiencies.* Westport, Conn., The AVI Publishing Co, 1983, p 43.
60. Ibid, pp 220-235.
61. Roe D: *Handbook: Interactions of Selected Drugs and Nutrients in Patients.* 3rd ed. Chicago, American Dietetic Association. 1982.
62. Rubinfeld Y: A progressive risk in serum copper levels in women taking oral contraceptives: A potential hazard? *Fertility and Sterility.* 1979; 32:599.
63. Adams P: Effect of pyridoxine hydrochloride (vitamin B_6) upon depression associated with oral contraceptives. *Lancet* 1973; 1:897.
64. Gross L, Brotman M: Hypoprothrombinemia and hemorrhage associated with cholestryamine therapy. *Ann Intern Med* 1970; 72:95.
65. Heaton K, Lever J, Barnard D: Osteomalacia associated with cholestryamine therapy for postileectomy diarrhea. *Gastroenterology.* 1972; 62:642.
66. Roe D: *Drug-Induced Nutritional Deficiencies.* Westport, Conn., The AVI Publishing Co, 1983, pp 133-134.
67. West R, Lloyd J: The effect of cholestyramine on intestinal absorption. *Gut* 1975; 16:93.
68. Mahan L, Krause M: *Food, Nutrition, and Diet Therapy* ed 7. Philadelphia, WB Saunders Co, 1984, pp 416-417.

69. Brown B, Albers J, Brunzell J: Normalization of elevated apolipoprotein-B with niacin plus colestipol in subjects with familiar combined hyperlipidemia. *Atherosclerosis* 1983; 3:A477.

70. Safer D, Allan R, Barr E,: Depression of growth in hyperactive children on stimulating drugs. *N Engl J Med* 1972; 287:217.

71. Garrison R, Somer E: *The Nutrition Desk Reference.* New Canaan, Conn., Keats Publishing Co, 1985, p 73.

72. Ibid, p 69.

73. Ibid, p 215-216.

74. Seelig M: Magnesium requirements in human nutrition. *Contemporary Nutrition* 1982; 7:1-2.

75. Garrison R, Somer E: *The Nutrition Desk Reference.* New Canaan, Conn., Keats Publishing Co, 1985, p 213.

76. Roe D: *Drug-Induced Nutritional Deficiencies.* Westport, Conn., The AVI Publishing Co, 1983, pp 27, 147.

77. Burrows M, Farr W: The action of mineral oil per se on the organism. *Proc Sco Exp Biol Med* 1927; 24:719.

78. Smith M, Spector H: Calcium and phosphorus metabolism in rats and dogs as influenced by the ingestion of mineral oil. *J Nutr.* 1940; 20:19.

79. Smith M, Spector H: Some effects on animal nutrition of the ingestion of mineral oil. *Univ Ariz Coll Agric Exper Sta Bull* 1940; 84:373.

80. Bidlack W, Smith C: The effect of nutritional factors on hepatic drug and toxicant metabolism. *J Amer Diet Assoc.* 1984; 84:892-898.

81. Neuvonen P, Gothoni G, Hackman R, et al: Interference of iron with the absorption of tetracyclines in man. *Br Med J* 1970; 4:532-534.

82. Roe D: *Drugs and Nutrition in the Geriatric Patient.* New York, Churchill Livingstone, 1984, pp 50-57.

83. Groves P, Schlesinger K: Introduction to biological psychology, ed 2. Dubuque, Iowa, Wm. C. Brown Co., 1982, pp 579-580,582.

84. Rosenzweig M, Leiman A: *Physiological Psychology.* Lexington, Mass, D.D.Heath and Co., 1982, pp 498,501.

85. Guyton A: *Textbook of Medical Physiology,* ed 5 Philadelphia, W.B. Saunders Co., 1976, p 741.

86. Kreiger D, Hughes J, (eds): *Neuroendocrinology.* Sunderland, Mass, Sinauer Assoc, Inc., 1980, p 170.

87. Roe D: *Drug-Induced Nutritional Deficiencies.* Westport, Conn., The AVI Publishing Co, 1983, p 122.

Glossary

Amino acid: A building block of protein; over 20 amino acids are used by the body to form proteins in hair, skin, blood, and other tissues.

Anorexia: The lack or loss of appetite for food, associated with weight loss and muscle wastage.

Antioxidant: A compound that protects other compounds or tissues from oxygen by itself reacting with oxygen.

Arrhythmia: Irregular heart beat.

Bacteria: Microscopic one-celled organisms found in food, the body, and all living matter; can contribute to both health and disease.

Bronchitis: Inflammation of the mucous membranes in the lungs.

Candidiasis: An infection by a fungus called candida; infection can be in lungs, heart, vagina, gastrointestinal tract, skin, nails, or other tissues.

Catabolism: The breakdown of substances in the body and the release of energy; example, glucose is catabolized to water, carbon dioxide and energy.

Cathartics: A medicine used to speed the movement of matter through the bowels.

Cholecystitis: Inflammation of the gall bladder.

Cirrhosis: Inflammation of fatty infiltration of the liver.

Dermatitis: Inflammation of the skin that is seen as a rash, sores, discoloration, eruptions, or ulcers.

Diuretic: An agent that increases the flow of urine.

Enzyme: A protein produced by the body that initiates and accelerates chemical reactions.

Estrogen: A female hormone; steroid hormone produced and secreted by the ovaries.

Free radical: A highly reactive compound derived from air pollution, radiation, cigarette smoke, or the incomplete breakdown of proteins and fats; reacts with fats in cell membranes and changes their shape or function.

Gastritis: Inflammation of the stomach.

Gastrointestinal: The stomach and intestinal tract.

Glucose: The building block of starch; sugar; blood sugar.

Hemorrhage: Seepage of blood from blood vessels into surrounding tissue

Hepatitis: Inflammation of the liver.

Hormone: A chemical substance produced by a group of cells or an organ, called an endocrine gland, that is released into the blood and transported to another organ or tissue, where it performs a specific action. ie.,insulin, estrogen, testosterone, adrenalin.

Hypertension: High blood pressure (hyper means "too much", tension means "pressure").

Insomnia: Chronic inability to sleep.

Jaundice: The appearance of bile in the blood.

Ketoacidosis: A condition where the body becomes too acidic with accompanying increase in ketone bodies in the blood.

Ketone bodies: A group of compounds, including acetone, that increase in the blood in diabetics and during fasting, starvation, preganancy, and other conditions.

Lactose intolerance: The inability to digest milk sugar (lactose) because of a deficiency of the digestive enzyme lactase.

Lethargy: Tired, sluggish, lack of energy.

Leukopenia: An abnormal reduction in white blood cells.

Neurotransmitters: A chemical that serves as a communication link between nerve cells or between a nerve cell and a muscle.

Obesity: Body weight more than 20% above desirable weight; excessive body fat.

Osteoporosis: Loss of calcium from the bone that results in reduced bone strength and increased fractures. The bones maintain the same diameter but become less dense.

Osteomalacia: Reduced deposition of calcium into bone tissue; one cause is a vitamin D deficiency.

Pancreas: The organ responsible for the production and secretion of numerous digestive enzymes and the hormone insulin responsible for the regulation of blood sugar.

Pancreatitis: Inflammation of the pancreas.

Platelets: Cell fragments in the blood that aid in blood coagulation.

Pneumonia: Inflammation of the lungs caused by a variety of bacteria and viruses.

Prophylactic: An agent that aids in the prevention of a disease.

Psoriasis: A chronic inflammation of the skin, especially on the scalp and body, characterized by the development of red patches covered by white scales.

Psychosis: Severe impairment of mental or emotional functions; a withdrawal from reality with an inability to test or evaluate reality correctly.

Rickets: Abnormal bone development caused by a vitamin D deficiency.

Seizures: The sudden onset of a disease or attack as in epileptic seizures; convulsions.

Steroid: A group of hormones formed from cholesterol or other sterols; includes the sex hormones (estrogen and testosterone) and the corticosteroids such as cortisone.

Testosterone: The male sex hormone; principal steroid hormone secreted by the testes.

Thrombocytopenia: An abnormal reduction in platelets.

Virus: Any of a large group of minute particles that are capable of infecting plants, animals, and humans.

Index

A

Achromycin (See Tetracycline)
Acne, p 44
Alcohol, p 1, 10, 21, 23, 27, 47, 48
  and folic acid, p 22, 43
  and magnesium, p 22, 41, 43
  and niacin, p 22
  and potassium, p 22
  and protein, p 23
  and sodium, p 22
  and vitamin B_1, p 21, 22, 43
  and vitamin B_2, p 12, 22
  and vitamin B_{12}, p 22, 43
  and vitamin C, p 22
  and zinc, p 21, 22, 43
Alcoholics, p 19
Aldactazide, p 61
Aldomet (See Methyldopa)
Aldoril, p 13, 61
Alophen (See Phenolphthalein)
Aluminum, p 20, 28
Amino Acids, p 18, 23, 29, 44
Amitriptyline, p 3, 30, 43
Amphetamines, p 5
Analgesics, p 21, 44
Anemia, p 22, 30, 42, 44, 45, 51
Antacids, p 20, 27, 47
  and alcohol, p 27
  and aluminum, p 27, 28
  and anemia, p 27
  and bone, p 27
  and calcium, p 27, 29
  and coffee, p 27
  and folic acid, p 27, 28, 47
  and iron, p 27, 29, 47
  and magnesium, p 27, 28
  and phosphate, p 22, 27, 28
  and sodium, p 28
  and vitamin A, p 47
  and vitamin B_{12}, p 27
Antibiotics, p 6, 11, 13, 41, 52, 53, 62
  and amino acids, p 29
  and calcium, p 29, 51
  and folic acid, p 29
  and gastrointestinal tract, p 29
  and influenza, p 28

  and iron, p 29, 51
  and magnesium, p 29, 41, 51
  and nitrogen, p 29
  and pneumonia, p 28
  and potassium, p 29
  and protein, p 29
  and sodium, p 29
  and tuberculosis, p 28
  and vitamin A, p 51
  and vitamin B_6, p 29
  and vitamin B_{12}, p 29
  and vitamin C, p 29
  and vitamin K, p 29
  and zinc, p 51
Anticoagulants, p 44, 52
Anticonvulsants, p 6, 29, 43, 62
  and anemia, p 30, 45
  and folic acid, p 30, 45
  and osteomalacia, p 29
  and rickets, p 29
  and vitamin B_1, p 43
  and vitamin B_6, p 45
  and vitamin B_{12}, p 30, 45
  and vitamin C, p 43
  and vitamin D, p 30, 43, 45
  and vitamin K, p 30
Antidepressants, p 3, 4, 6, 30, 54
  and B vitamins, p 31
  and calcium, p 31, 43
  and magnesium, p 31, 43
  and vitamin C, p 31
Antifungal, p 4, 5, 43
  and potassium, p 43
  and magnesium, p 43
  and nitrogen, p 43
Antihistamines, p 3, 43
Anti-inflammatory, p 13, 22, 43
  and alcohol, p 48
  and carotene, p 43
  and folic acid, p 32, 49
  and iron, p 22
  and potassium, p 43
  and sodium, p 43
  and vitamin B_{12}, p 43
Antimicrobial, p 43, 45
  and calcium, p 46
  and potassium, p 45, 46
  and vitamin B_2, p 43

70

71